GAST[illegible] DIET PLANS MADE SIMPLE

The Perfect Guide On Gastric Bypass Meal Plans Including Food To Eat And Avoid Plus Diet Before And After Gastric Bypass Surgery

Clifford Riggins

TABLE OF CONTENT

CHAPTER 1

TABLE OF CONTENT

Gastric bypass surgery is a lifesaving procedure. You will get in shape. You will diminish your co-morbidities. You will feel good and look better. Be that as it may, to be effective (long haul), you need to change your diet.

This healthys straightforward, yet it's definitely not. Be set up for a battle. You've consumed a lot of your time on building and strengthening terrible diet. Those need to change.

Realizing what you can and can't eat is the initial move towards a healthy eating routine. Your diet for the initial five weeks after gastric bypass medical procedure is significant for two reasons.

Your safety. Eating an inappropriate food could disturb your healing stomach.

Resetting your awful diet and supplanting them with new healthy habits.

CHAPTER 2

STAGES OF GASTRIC BYPASS

Pre-Op Liquid Diet

So as to lessen the measure of fat around the liver and spleen, a preoperative fluid eating routine must be followed 7-14 days before gastric bypass medical procedure. In the event that this diet isn't followed, at that point medical procedure might be postponed or dropped intra-operatively (during the procedure).

I can't pressure enough that it is so critical to follow the pre-operation diet. Follow your pre-operation diet.

Food diary and water.A enormous liver keeps your specialist from imagining certain life systems during the methodology. In the event that the liver is excessively enormous, it at that point gets hazardous to play out your gastric bypass medical procedure. Medical procedure may then be dropped and rescheduled to a later date.

The 1-multi week pre-operation diet will incorporate the accompanying components:

Protein shakes or dinner substitution shakes will be the diet's essential part.

Just without sugar refreshments are permitted (sugar substitutes are alright).

No stimulated or carbonated refreshments are allowed.

Soup stock with no strong bits of food might be devoured.

V8 and vegetable juice are worthy.

Amazingly dainty cream of wheat or cream of rice may likewise be eaten.

A couple of every day servings of lean meat or potentially vegetables may be alright, yet just in the event that they are endorsed by your specialist or enrolled dietician.

All drinks and fluids ought to be tasted gradually. Drinks ought not be overwhelmed by suppers, and the patient should hold up at any rate 30 minutes after a feast before devouring any kind of fluid.

Isolating your fluids and solids applies post-operatively (after medical procedure) yet it's a decent propensity to begin pre-operatively.

An every day supper plan for the patient's pre-operation fluid eating routine may resemble this:

Pre-employable example feast plan table.

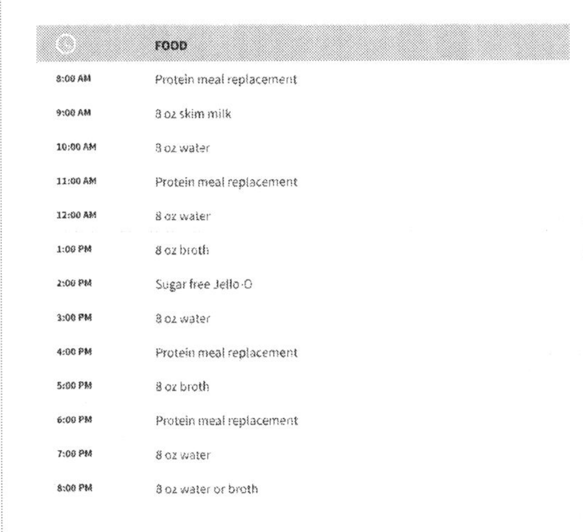

🕐	FOOD
8:00 AM	Protein meal replacement
9:00 AM	8 oz skim milk
10:00 AM	8 oz water
11:00 AM	Protein meal replacement
12:00 AM	8 oz water
1:00 PM	8 oz broth
2:00 PM	Sugar free Jello-O
3:00 PM	8 oz water
4:00 PM	Protein meal replacement
5:00 PM	8 oz broth
6:00 PM	Protein meal replacement
7:00 PM	8 oz water
8:00 PM	8 oz water or broth

High Protein Meal Replacements

During the pre-operation stage (preceding medical procedure) your body will go into ketosis. This permits your body to utilize your fat stores as a vitality source. The outcome is the fat in your liver psychologists extensively in a short measure of time. As observed over, your diet is high in protein and low in sugars. The following are some proposed high protein supper substitutions:

Notes Pre-Op

Converse with your PCP about halting certain drugs before medical procedure. The accompanying prescriptions are commonly halted multi week before medical procedure and may require tightening the portion.

Coumadin

Steroids

Other enemy of coagulation prescriptions

Headache medicine, Motrin, Advil, Celebrex, and some other NSAIDs

Substitution hormones

Anti-conception medication

if you have rest apnea and utilize a CPAP machine, plan on carrying it to the emergency clinic. Buy nutrients and enhancements ahead of time of medical procedure. Locate a decent protein shake.

In the event that you smoke you should stop preceding medical procedure. Smoker's have an expanded danger of blood clusters and confusions during and after medical procedure. Make an arrangement and execute it half a month preceding medical procedure.

Oppose the "Last Supper Syndrome." A vacant stomach is simpler to work with.

Try not to eat or drink anything upon the arrival of medical procedure (normally, beginning at 12 PM the prior night).

CHAPTER 3

Post-Op Dietary Guidelines

When gastric bypass medical procedure is finished, a severe post-operation diet plan should be followed. There is presently a staple line in your stomach that must be permitted to recuperate. Certain foods can upset the mending procedure, put undue weight on the staple line, and lead to a hole.

The eating routine for a post-operation gastric bypass quiet comprises of four phases:

Table indicating 4 phases of gastric bypass diet

Week 1 – Clear Liquids

STAGE ONE	STAGE TWO	STAGE THREE	STAGE FOUR
Clear Liquids	Pureed Foods	Soft Foods	Solid Foods
Estimated duration	**Estimated duration**	**Estimated duration**	**Estimated duration**
1 to 7 days immediately after surgery	Approximately 14 days after stage one is completed	2 weeks up to 2 months after stage two is completed	For the remainder of the patient's lifetime

For one to seven days after gastric bypass medical process, just clear fluids are to be increased at the pace of 1 to 2 ounces for every hour. The patient's dietitian will choose to what extent this stage will last and propose dietary rules.

Clear fluids suggested by the dietitian will most likely incorporate the accompanying things:

water

sans fat milk

sans fat stock

sans sugar Jello

A phase one clear fluid utilization calendar may resemble this:

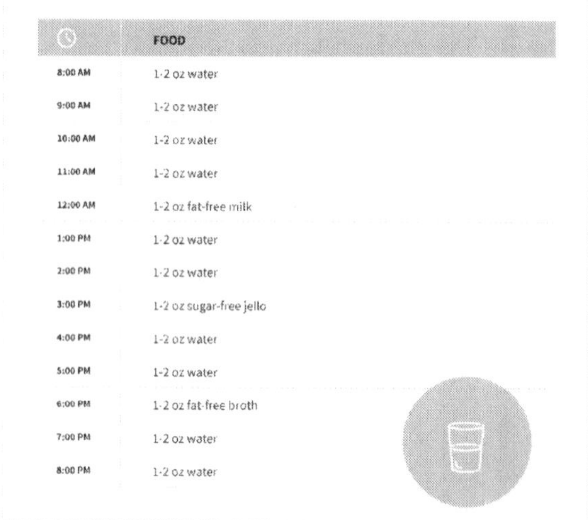

	FOOD
8:00 AM	1-2 oz water
9:00 AM	1-2 oz water
10:00 AM	1-2 oz water
11:00 AM	1-2 oz water
12:00 AM	1-2 oz fat-free milk
1:00 PM	1-2 oz water
2:00 PM	1-2 oz water
3:00 PM	1-2 oz sugar-free jello
4:00 PM	1-2 oz water
5:00 PM	1-2 oz water
6:00 PM	1-2 oz fat-free broth
7:00 PM	1-2 oz water
8:00 PM	1-2 oz water

Clear fluid, stage 1 gastric bypass diet plan.

During this stage, it's critical to remain hydrated. A few specialists may need you to begin protein shakes a couple of days after medical procedure. Follow your specialist's rules.

Week Two and Three – Pureed Foods and Protein Shakes

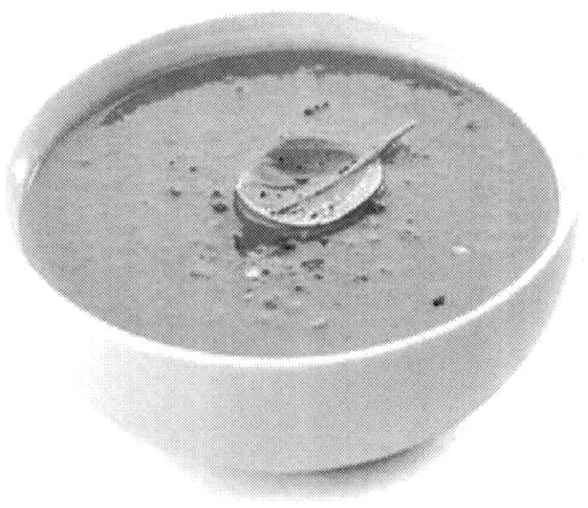

Following 1 to 7 days of drinking clear fluids, you will be offered consent to devour condensed wellsprings of protein. This phase of the post-operation diet will normally keep going for multi week (infrequently 2).

Due to the patient's littler stomach size, the individual ought to have a few littler suppers for the duration of the day. Your every day admission ought to be around 60-70 grams of (protein shakes, egg whites, pureed meat/fish) and roughly 64 ounces (around 8 glasses) of clear fluids (as characterized in stage one) not including the liquid in the pureed foods.

Pureed food.Caffeinated and carbonated refreshments ought

to are not to be devoured. Refined sugars and basic starches (counting sugar liquor) ought to be dodged also.

The following is a rundown of the pureed protein sources that are normally permitted by the patient's dietitian or specialist:

Protein shakes

Egg whites

Non-fat delicate cheddar

Non-fat curds

These food substances ought to be pureed with water, without fat milk, or sans fat stock. Clear fluids (water) ought not be expended simultaneously as the pureed foods. As a general rule, it is normally recommended that the patient not drink any unmistakable fluid 30 minutes before a feast and an hour after a dinner.

Clear fluids ought to be tasted gradually, and straws ought not be utilized ifthey may carry undesirable air into the stomach.

It is important to take a couple of multivitamins (containing iron) each day so as to forestall supplement deficiencies. The multivitamins should be in chewable or fluid structure.

It is additionally critical to enhance your eating routine with calcium citrate; the suggested sum will ordinarily be a few dosages with each portion running from 400 mg to 600 mg. Calcium citrate supplementation ought to be isolated from the multivitamin measurements by in any event two hours. This is on the grounds that iron and calcium can meddle with every others ingestion.

A phase two feast plan may resemble this:

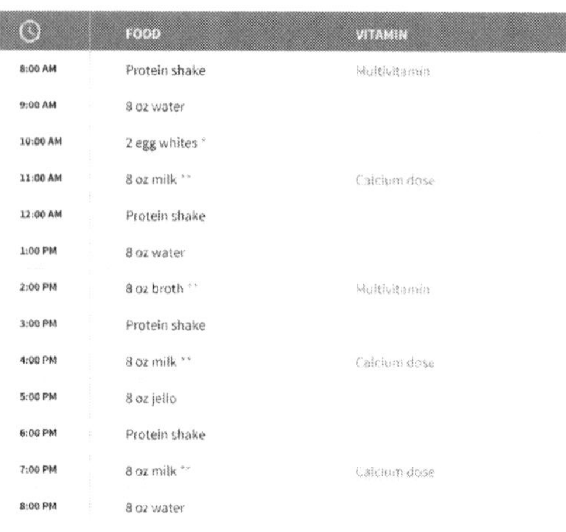

	FOOD	VITAMIN
8:00 AM	Protein shake	Multivitamin
9:00 AM	8 oz water	
10:00 AM	2 egg whites *	
11:00 AM	8 oz milk **	Calcium dose
12:00 AM	Protein shake	
1:00 PM	8 oz water	
2:00 PM	8 oz broth **	Multivitamin
3:00 PM	Protein shake	
4:00 PM	8 oz milk **	Calcium dose
5:00 PM	8 oz jello	
6:00 PM	Protein shake	
7:00 PM	8 oz milk **	Calcium dose
8:00 PM	8 oz water	

Stage 2 gastric bypass diet

Week 4 and 5 – Soft Foods

This phase of the diet will take into account an extremely steady reintroduction of delicate foods into your eating routine. This stage ordinarily keeps going around 1 or fourteen days.

This bit of the eating routine will incorporate delicate meats and cooked vegetables.

The supplement objectives will continue as before as in stage two. 60-70 grams of protein and 64 ounces of liquid is suggested day by day. The serving size of protein in stage three ought to be around 1 to 2 ounces and you'll likely have 3 to 6 little dinners.

Stage three, similar to arrange two, centers around excellent lean protein sources.

While stage 3 keeps on concentrating on top notch lean protein sources, up to three servings of delicate vegetables may likewise be permitted; a minuscule bit of fat may likewise be allowed (this little part of fat will most likely be from a solitary serving of ready avocado).

Proposals for the protein sources in this phase of the diet will most likely incorporate a few of the accompanying things:

Meat, Dairy, and Eggs

lean chicken

lean turkey

fish

egg whites

non-fat curds

non-fat cheddar

tofu

Vegetables

potatoes

carrots

green beans

tomatoes

squash

cucumbers

bananas

avocados

You will at present need two multivitamins and a few 400-600 mg portions of calcium citrate (with every one of these dosages to be dismantled at any rate two hours from one another).

Your dietitian may suggest you take 1,000 IU of Vitamin D3 every day; this will no doubt be isolated into two 500 IU portions. These ought to be taken with your calcium citrate. Likewise, a day by day portion of sublingual B12 (500-1,000 mcg) might be suggested. A week after week or month to month infusion or intranasal choice might be accessible for B12. A few dietitians may need you to start nutrient D3 and B12 supplementation in stage two.

This is the thing that a run of the mill stage three dinner plan may resemble:

	FOOD	VITAMIN
8:00 AM	4 scrambled egg white	Multivitamin
9:00 AM	8 oz water	Sublingual B12
10:00 AM	1/4 cup non-fat cottage cheese	
11:00 AM	8 oz skim milk	Calcium dose & Vitamin D
12:00 AM	2 oz tuna - 1/2 cup carrots **	
1:00 PM	8 oz vegetable juice	
2:00 PM	8 oz chicken broth	Multivitamin
3:00 PM	2 oz chicken * - 1 tbsp avocado **	
4:00 PM	8 oz skim milk	Calcium dose
5:00 PM	2 oz turkey * - 1/2 cup potatoes ****	
6:00 PM	8 oz water	
7:00 PM	8 oz skim milk	Calcium dose & Vitamin D
8:00 PM	8 oz water	

Week 6 – Solid Foods

Strong food is back! You've made it this far and it's a great opportunity to begin eating genuine food. This doesn't mean you get the opportunity to eat anything you desire.

Gastric bypass food pyramid.A diet comprising of protein, vegetables, a restricted measure of grains, and practically nothing, assuming any, refined sugars ought to be followed for a mind-blowing remainder.

Tips for beginning strong foods:

Present each new food in turn; in a perfect world not more than one new food daily so you can measure your body's response.

Eat gradually. Bite your food well, 15 seconds each chomp. Utilize the clock on the Baritastic application.

Separate your food and water by at any rate 30 minutes.

Keep on drinking in any event 64 ounces of water a day.

Eat your protein first, vegetables second and sugars third (in a perfect world solid grains and additionally natural products, not prepared foods).

Eat genuine supplement thick foods. Avoid pre-bundled and handled foods with a ton of fixings.

Understand marks. Concentrate on foods low in starches and a calorie to protein proportion of 10 to 1 or less (add a zero to the grams of protein and in the event that the complete calories are more than that, at that point you might need to maintain a strategic distance from that food – especially in the event that you are battling to arrive at your protein objectives).

Dumping disorder happens when sweet as well as greasy foods have been expended too rapidly or in too huge an amount. The stomach dumps the food into the small digestive tract before it's appropriately separated. Dumping disorder for the most part causes sickness, squeezing, loose bowels, perspiring, regurgitating, or an expansion in pulse; these side effects as a rule wear off following a couple of hours. Be that as it may, the experience of 'dumping' is upsetting and you'll need to stay away from it.

To diminish the danger of dumping:

Stay away from high sugar/refined starch foods.

Eat gradually.

Bite your food well.

Certain foods are extremely hard to process and ought to be drawn closer with alert:

meat

pork

shellfish

grapes

nuts

entire grains

corn

beans

Essentially, similar rules found in stage three will be extended into this fourth and last phase of the patient's post-operation dietary arrangement. The protein consumption, nutrient supplementation, and clear fluid prerequisites continue as before.

More foods grown from the ground (both cooked and crude) may now be deliberately added to your diet. Limited quantities of fat and exceptionally modest quantities of sugar may now be included with alert. Carbonated and juiced refreshments may now be devoured with some restraint.

The all out caloric admission every day will normally extend from 800 to 1,200 and up to 1,500 year and a half after medical procedure.

A phase four dinner plan would resemble this:

	FOOD	VITAMIN
8:00 AM	2 scrambled eggs - 1 piece of toast (lightly buttered)	Multivitamin
9:00 AM	8 oz water	Sublingual B12
10:00 AM	1 cup low-fat yoghurt, Protein Shake	
11:00 AM	8 oz skim milk	Calcium dose & Vitamin D
12:00 AM	8 oz water	
1:00 PM	2 oz dark chicken - 1/2 cup steamed carrots	
2:00 PM	8 oz decaffeinated tea	Multivitamin
3:00 PM	8 oz chicken soup w/small pieces of meat and vegetables	
4:00 PM	8 oz skim milk	Calcium dose
5:00 PM	8 oz water	
6:00 PM	2 oz fish - 1 baked potato (with a few toppings)	
7:00 PM	8 oz skim milk	Calcium dose & Vitamin D
8:00 PM	8 oz water (optional)	

CHAPTER 4

Physical Activity And Exercise

It's an ideal opportunity to begin working out. As a matter of fact, you ought to have begun in front of an audience 2. Strolling, running, biking, weight lifting, high impact exercise, kayaking, badminton, climbing, and moving in your room like an insane individual would all be able to be added to your week by week schedule. Guarantee that you are getting at any rate 30 minutes of activity 5 to 7 days every week. It doesn't make a difference how you do it, do what needs to be done.

Note: Do not lift in excess of 10 pounds for at any rate a month and a half after medical procedure. This can squeeze your inside fastens and result in a hernia.

CHAPTER 5

Picking Gastric Bypass Appropriate Foods

When all is said in done, you'll need to pick foods that are high to direct in protein, low in starches and moderate in great fats.

foods with great (solid) fats include:

avocados

salmon

nuts

sardines

nut margarines

coconut oil

General rules include:

Pick lean meats.

Canned fish and salmon.

Stay away from oily and fiery foods.

Stay away from entire milk.

Eat supplement thick foods (entire organic products, vegetables, meats, eggs).

Plan your dinners.

Include your family in good dieting choices.

Shop for healthy foods.

Restrict or kill sweets.

Try not to entice yourself with a wash room loaded with low quality foods.

Take out inexpensive food.

Eat out just once in a while.

Take quality dietary enhancements/nutrients.

Separate your water and food by in any event 30 minutes.

Present new foods gradually.

Every supper ought to be no bigger than your clench hand.

CHAPTER 6

CONCLUSION

Gastric bypass is one of the most secure and best types of weight reduction medical procedure. Therefore, it is frequently alluded to as the "highest quality level."

You will get more fit with gastric bypass medical procedure – on normal 70% of your overabundance weight. Be that as it may, it's dependent upon you to keep the weight off.

Follow your specialist's eating routine rules, practice 5 to 7 times each week for at any rate 30 minutes, and pick supplement thick non-prepared foods. You will keep the weight off, lessen drugs, become more advantageous, and carry on with a more drawn out, more joyful life.

THE END

Made in the USA
Coppell, TX
11 June 2021